MW00915054

Slow Cooker Dog Food Cookbook

Easy Nutrient-Packed Recipes to Support Your Furry
Friend's Health, Energy, and Happiness at Every Stage
of Life

Nora Howland

Nimbus Press Concepts

Contents

Introduction

Why Homemade Dog Food?

As pet parents, we all want the best for our furry companions. Their health, happiness, and well-being are often at the forefront of our minds. One way to ensure that your dog is getting the very best is by taking control of their diet, and what better way to do this than by preparing homemade meals? In recent years, there has been a growing awareness of the benefits of homemade dog food. More and more pet owners are turning away from commercial dog food and embracing the idea of making meals for their dogs at home.

But why homemade dog food? There are several compelling reasons to consider this approach. Firstly, homemade dog food allows you to know exactly what your dog is eating. You have full control over the ingredients, ensuring that your dog's meals are free from harmful additives, preservatives, and fillers commonly found in commercial dog foods. This is particularly important for dogs with food allergies or sensitivities, as you can tailor their diet to avoid specific ingredients.

Another significant advantage of homemade dog food is the ability to provide fresh, whole foods that are rich in nutrients. While commercial dog food is convenient, it often lacks the nutritional value that fresh, home-prepared meals can offer. By using wholesome ingredients like lean meats, vegetables, and whole grains, you can create balanced meals that support your dog's overall health and vitality.

Moreover, homemade dog food allows for customization based on your dog's specific needs. Whether your dog requires a special diet for weight management, joint health, or digestive issues, you can create meals that cater to these needs. This level of personalization is difficult to achieve with commercial dog food, where one size rarely fits all.

Of course, there's also the simple joy of cooking for your dog. Preparing meals for your dog can strengthen the bond between you and your pet, making mealtime a special occasion for both of you. The love and care you put into making their food can contribute to their overall happiness and well-being.

Understanding Your Dog's Nutritional Needs

Before diving into homemade dog food, it's crucial to understand your dog's nutritional needs. Dogs, like humans, require a balanced diet to thrive. This means that their meals need to include the right amounts of proteins, fats, carbohydrates, vitamins, and minerals. However, unlike humans, dogs have specific dietary requirements that must be met to maintain their health.

Proteins are the building blocks of your dog's body. They are essential for growth, muscle development, and tissue repair. High-quality animal proteins, such as chicken, beef, and fish, should be a staple in your dog's diet. These proteins provide the essential amino acids that your dog's body cannot produce on its own.

Fats are another important component of your dog's diet. They provide a concentrated source of energy and are necessary for healthy skin and coat. Fats also help with the absorption of fat-soluble vitamins, such as A, D, E, and K. While fats are essential, it's important to provide them in moderation to prevent obesity and other health issues.

Carbohydrates provide energy and are a source of fiber, which aids in digestion. While dogs do not have a strict dietary requirement for carbohydrates, including them in moderation can be beneficial, especially for active dogs. Whole grains, like brown rice and oats, and vegetables, such as sweet potatoes and carrots, are excellent sources of healthy carbohydrates.

Vitamins and minerals are crucial for your dog's overall health and well-being. They play a role in everything from bone health to immune function. For example, calcium and phosphorus are important for bone development, while vitamins A and E support skin health and immune function. When preparing homemade dog food, it's essential to ensure that your dog is getting the right balance of these nutrients, either through food or supplements.

If your dog has specific dietary needs, such as allergies, sensitivities, or medical conditions, it's essential to tailor their diet accordingly. For example, dogs with food allergies may need to avoid certain proteins or grains, while dogs with kidney disease may require a diet low in phosphorus. Consulting with a veterinarian or a veterinary nutritionist can help you create a diet plan that meets your dog's unique needs.

Lastly, always consult with your veterinarian before making any significant changes to your dog's diet. While homemade dog food offers many benefits, it's essential to ensure that your dog's meals are balanced and meet their nutritional needs. Your vet can help you determine the right portions, ingredients, and supplements for your dog's specific health requirements.

Using a Slow Cooker for Dog Food

One of the best tools for preparing homemade dog food is a slow cooker. Slow cookers are incredibly convenient, allowing you to prepare nutritious meals with minimal effort. With a slow cooker, you can simply add your ingredients, set the timer, and let it do the work for you. This is especially useful for busy pet parents who want to provide homemade meals without spending hours in the kitchen.

Using a slow cooker also has several benefits for your dog's food. The slow cooking process preserves the nutrients in the ingredients, ensuring that your dog gets the maximum nutritional value from their meals. Unlike high-heat cooking methods, slow cooking retains the vitamins and minerals in the food, making it a healthier option for your dog.

Another advantage of slow cooking is that it allows the flavors to develop over time, making the food more palatable for your dog. Even picky eaters are likely to enjoy the rich, savory flavors that slow-cooked meals offer. Plus, the tender texture of slow-cooked food is easy for dogs to chew and digest, making it a great option for dogs of all ages, especially seniors with dental issues.

When choosing a slow cooker, consider the size and features that will best suit your needs. A larger slow cooker is ideal if you're preparing meals in bulk or have multiple dogs. Look for a slow cooker with a timer and a keep-warm function, which will allow you to set it and forget it while ensuring that the food stays warm until you're ready to serve it.

Safety is also an important consideration when using a slow cooker for dog food. Always ensure that the food reaches a safe internal temperature to prevent the growth of harmful bacteria. Avoid using ingredients that are toxic to dogs, such as onions, garlic, and certain spices. It's also important to store any leftovers in the refrigerator or freezer promptly to prevent spoilage.

In the following chapters, we'll explore a variety of slow cooker recipes tailored to meet your dog's specific needs. From nutrient-rich meals for puppies to easy-to-digest options for seniors, these recipes will help you provide wholesome, homemade meals that your dog will love.

Chapter One

Puppy Power: Recipes for Growing Dogs

Puppy Protein Stew

Ingredients:
- 1 lb lean ground turkey
- 1 cup quinoa, rinsed
- 1 cup chopped carrots
- 1 cup chopped spinach
- 1/2 cup peas
- 4 cups low-sodium chicken broth
- 1 tbsp olive oil

Instructions:
1. Heat the olive oil in a skillet over medium heat. Add the ground turkey and cook until browned.
2. Transfer the turkey to the slow cooker.
3. Add the quinoa, carrots, spinach, peas, and chicken broth.
4. Stir to combine, then cover and cook on low for 4-5 hours.
5. Allow the stew to cool before serving to your puppy.

Chicken and Brown Rice Puppy Delight

Ingredients:
- 1 lb boneless, skinless chicken breasts, diced
- 1 cup brown rice, rinsed
- 1 cup chopped broccoli
- 1/2 cup chopped sweet potato
- 1/4 cup chopped apples (core and seeds removed)
- 4 cups water

Instructions:
1. Place all ingredients in the slow cooker.
2. Stir to combine.
3. Cover and cook on low for 6-8 hours, until the chicken is fully cooked and the rice is tender.
4. Let it cool before serving.

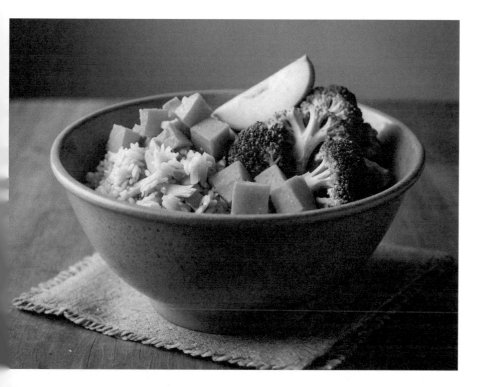

Puppy Pot Roast

Ingredients:
- 1 lb beef stew meat, cut into small pieces
- 1 cup barley
- 1 cup diced carrots
- 1/2 cup diced celery
- 1/2 cup green beans, chopped
- 4 cups low-sodium beef broth

Instructions:
1. Place the beef stew meat, barley, carrots, celery, and green beans in the slow cooker.
2. Pour in the beef broth.
3. Stir to combine and cover.
4. Cook on low for 6-7 hours, until the beef is tender and the barley is fully cooked.
5. Cool before serving.

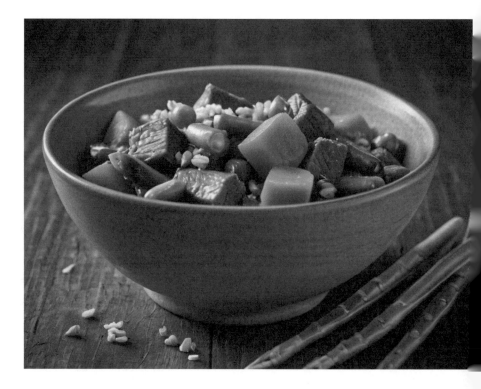

Salmon and Sweet Potato Puppy Feast

Ingredients:
- 2 salmon fillets, skin removed, diced
- 1 cup diced sweet potatoes
- 1/2 cup chopped zucchini
- 1/2 cup chopped green beans
- 1/4 cup blueberries
- 4 cups water

Instructions:
1. Place all ingredients in the slow cooker.
2. Stir to combine.
3. Cover and cook on low for 4-5 hours.
4. Once cooked, allow the food to cool.
5. Mash the mixture slightly before serving to make it easier for puppies to eat.

Turkey and Pumpkin Puppy Stew

Ingredients:
- 1 lb ground turkey
- 1 cup canned pumpkin (pure, unsweetened)
- 1/2 cup diced carrots
- 1/2 cup chopped green beans
- 1/4 cup chopped parsley
- 4 cups low-sodium chicken broth

Instructions:
1. Brown the ground turkey in a skillet over medium heat.
2. Transfer the turkey to the slow cooker.
3. Add the pumpkin, carrots, green beans, parsley, and chicken broth.
4. Stir to combine and cover.
5. Cook on low for 4-5 hours.
6. Cool before serving.

Puppy Chicken and Oatmeal Breakfast

Ingredients:
- 1 lb boneless, skinless chicken thighs, diced
- 1 cup steel-cut oats
- 1/2 cup diced apples (core and seeds removed)
- 1/2 cup chopped carrots
- 1/4 cup cranberries
- 4 cups low-sodium chicken broth

Instructions:
1. Place all ingredients in the slow cooker.
2. Stir to combine.
3. Cover and cook on low for 5-6 hours, until the chicken is cooked through and the oats are tender.
4. Let it cool before serving.

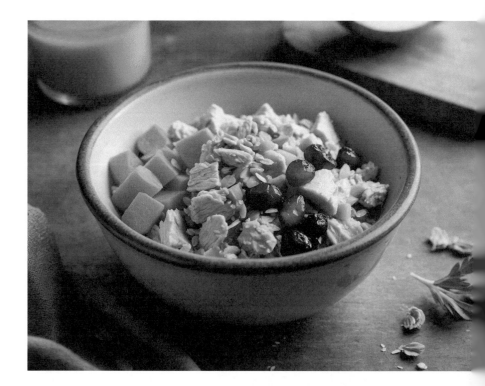

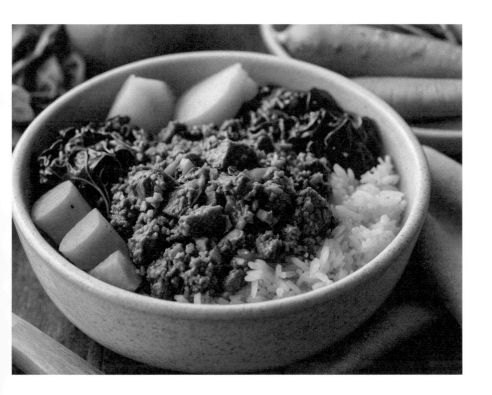

Lamb and Rice Puppy Chow

Ingredients:
- 1 lb ground lamb
- 1 cup white rice, rinsed
- 1/2 cup chopped spinach
- 1/2 cup diced carrots
- 1/4 cup chopped pears (core and seeds removed)
- 4 cups water

Instructions:
1. Place all ingredients in the slow cooker.
2. Stir to combine.
3. Cover and cook on low for 5-6 hours, until the lamb is cooked and the rice is tender.
4. Allow to cool before serving.

Beef and Veggie Puppy Casserole

Ingredients:
- 1 lb lean ground beef
- 1 cup chopped zucchini
- 1/2 cup chopped butternut squash
- 1/2 cup peas
- 1/4 cup chopped parsley
- 4 cups low-sodium beef broth

Instructions:
1. Brown the ground beef in a skillet over medium heat.
2. Transfer the beef to the slow cooker.
3. Add the zucchini, squash, peas, parsley, and beef broth.
4. Stir to combine and cover.
5. Cook on low for 6-7 hours.
6. Cool before serving.

Chicken and Quinoa Puppy Stew

Ingredients:
- 1 lb boneless, skinless chicken breasts, diced
- 1 cup quinoa, rinsed
- 1/2 cup chopped kale
- 1/2 cup diced sweet potatoes
- 1/4 cup diced apples (core and seeds removed)
- 4 cups water

Instructions:
1. Place all ingredients in the slow cooker.
2. Stir to combine.
3. Cover and cook on low for 6-7 hours, until the chicken is fully cooked and the quinoa is tender.
4. Let it cool before serving.

Fish and Rice Puppy Meal

Ingredients:
- 2 cod fillets, skin removed, diced
- 1 cup white rice, rinsed
- 1/2 cup chopped broccoli
- 1/2 cup diced carrots
- 1/4 cup chopped parsley
- 4 cups water

Instructions:
1. Place all ingredients in the slow cooker.
2. Stir to combine.
3. Cover and cook on low for 4-5 hours, until the fish is cooked and the rice is tender.
4. Cool before serving.

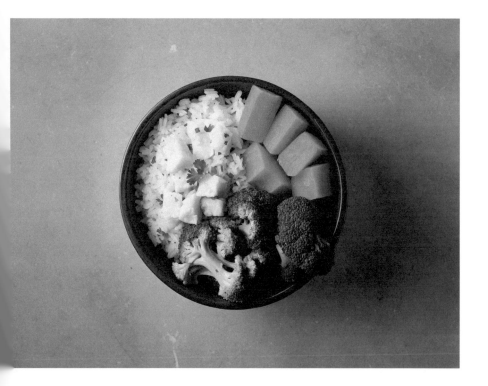

These recipes are designed to provide a variety of nutrients essential for a growing puppy, focusing on lean proteins, healthy grains, and vegetables. They are easy to prepare using a slow cooker, ensuring that your puppy enjoys nutritious and delicious meals without much hassle.

Chapter Two

Adult Dog Essentials: Everyday Meals

Beef and Brown Rice Daily Delight

Ingredients:
- 1 lb lean ground beef
- 1 cup brown rice, rinsed
- 1 cup chopped carrots
- 1/2 cup peas
- 1/4 cup chopped parsley
- 4 cups low-sodium beef broth

Instructions:
1. Brown the ground beef in a skillet over medium heat.
2. Transfer the beef to the slow cooker.
3. Add the brown rice, carrots, peas, parsley, and beef broth.
4. Stir to combine.
5. Cover and cook on low for 6-7 hours, until the rice is tender and the flavors are well-blended.
6. Let it cool before serving.

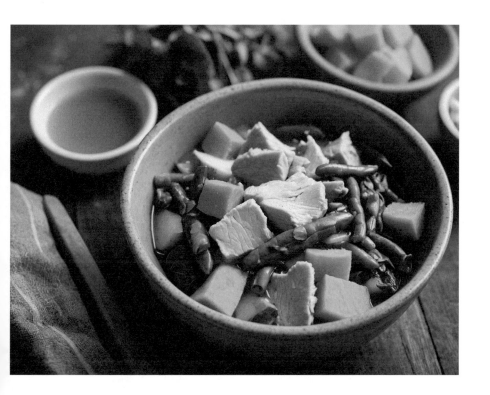

Chicken and Sweet Potato Hearty Meal

Ingredients:
- 1 lb boneless, skinless chicken thighs, diced
- 1 cup diced sweet potatoes
- 1/2 cup chopped green beans
- 1/2 cup chopped spinach
- 1/4 cup chopped apples (core and seeds removed)
- 4 cups low-sodium chicken broth

Instructions:
1. Place all ingredients in the slow cooker.
2. Stir to combine.
3. Cover and cook on low for 6-8 hours, until the chicken is tender and the sweet potatoes are soft.
4. Allow the food to cool before serving.

Turkey and Oats Balanced Bowl

Ingredients:
- 1 lb ground turkey
- 1 cup rolled oats
- 1/2 cup diced carrots
- 1/2 cup chopped zucchini
- 1/4 cup cranberries
- 4 cups water

Instructions:
1. Brown the ground turkey in a skillet over medium heat.
2. Transfer the turkey to the slow cooker.
3. Add the oats, carrots, zucchini, cranberries, and water.
4. Stir to combine and cover.
5. Cook on low for 5-6 hours, until the oats are tender and the flavors are well-combined.
6. Cool before serving.

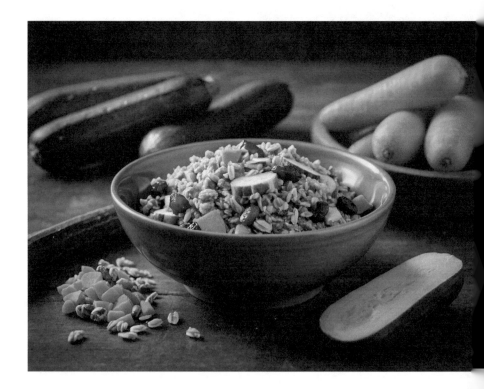

Fish and Vegetable Medley

Ingredients:
- 2 white fish fillets (such as cod or tilapia), skin removed, diced
- 1 cup diced carrots
- 1/2 cup chopped green beans
- 1/2 cup chopped sweet potatoes
- 1/4 cup chopped parsley
- 4 cups water

Instructions:
1. Place all ingredients in the slow cooker.
2. Stir to combine.
3. Cover and cook on low for 4-5 hours, until the fish is cooked and the vegetables are tender.
4. Let it cool before serving.

Lamb and Barley Dinner

Ingredients:
- 1 lb ground lamb
- 1 cup barley
- 1/2 cup chopped broccoli
- 1/2 cup chopped carrots
- 1/4 cup chopped apples (core and seeds removed)
- 4 cups low-sodium chicken broth

Instructions:
1. Place all ingredients in the slow cooker.
2. Stir to combine.
3. Cover and cook on low for 6-7 hours, until the barley is tender and the lamb is fully cooked.
4. Cool before serving.

Chicken and Quinoa Power Meal

Ingredients:
- 1 lb boneless, skinless chicken breasts, diced
- 1 cup quinoa, rinsed
- 1/2 cup chopped kale
- 1/2 cup diced carrots
- 1/4 cup blueberries
- 4 cups water

Instructions:
1. Place all ingredients in the slow cooker.
2. Stir to combine.
3. Cover and cook on low for 6-7 hours, until the quinoa is tender and the chicken is fully cooked.
4. Let it cool before serving.

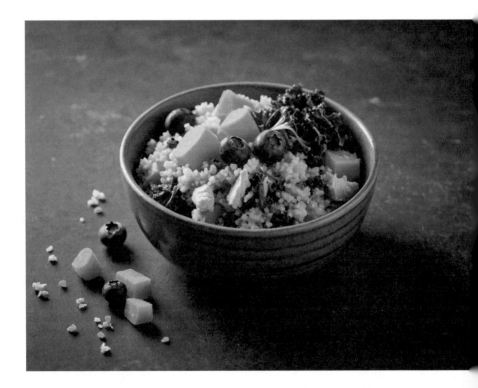

Beef and Pumpkin Feast

Ingredients:
- 1 lb lean ground beef
- 1 cup canned pumpkin (pure, unsweetened)
- 1/2 cup diced carrots
- 1/2 cup chopped green beans
- 1/4 cup chopped parsley
- 4 cups low-sodium beef broth

Instructions:
1. Brown the ground beef in a skillet over medium heat.
2. Transfer the beef to the slow cooker.
3. Add the pumpkin, carrots, green beans, parsley, and beef broth.
4. Stir to combine.
5. Cover and cook on low for 5-6 hours, until the flavors are well-blended and the vegetables are tender.
6. Cool before serving.

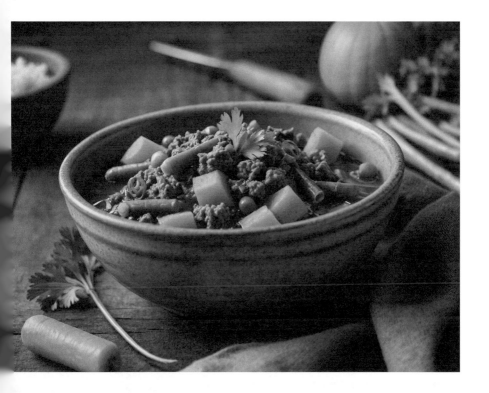

Turkey and Lentil Nourishing Stew

Ingredients:
- 1 lb ground turkey
- 1 cup lentils, rinsed
- 1/2 cup chopped carrots
- 1/2 cup chopped zucchini
- 1/4 cup cranberries
- 4 cups low-sodium chicken broth

Instructions:
1. Brown the ground turkey in a skillet over medium heat.
2. Transfer the turkey to the slow cooker.
3. Add the lentils, carrots, zucchini, cranberries, and chicken broth.
4. Stir to combine.
5. Cover and cook on low for 6-8 hours, until the lentils are tender and the flavors are well-combined.
6. Let it cool before serving.

Salmon and Sweet Potato Dinner

Ingredients:
- 2 salmon fillets, skin removed, diced
- 1 cup diced sweet potatoes
- 1/2 cup chopped spinach
- 1/2 cup chopped green beans
- 1/4 cup blueberries
- 4 cups water

Instructions:
1. Place all ingredients in the slow cooker.
2. Stir to combine.
3. Cover and cook on low for 4-5 hours, until the salmon is cooked and the sweet potatoes are tender.
4. Cool before serving.

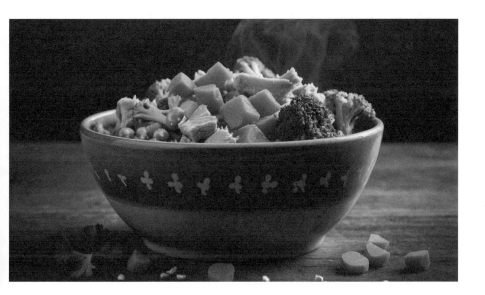

Chicken and Vegetable Classic

Ingredients:
- 1 lb boneless, skinless chicken thighs, diced
- 1 cup chopped broccoli
- 1/2 cup chopped carrots
- 1/2 cup peas
- 1/4 cup chopped parsley
- 4 cups low-sodium chicken broth

Instructions:
1. Place all ingredients in the slow cooker.
2. Stir to combine.
3. Cover and cook on low for 6-7 hours, until the chicken is tender and the vegetables are cooked through.
4. Allow the food to cool before serving.

These recipes provide balanced and nutritious meals for adult dogs, focusing on lean proteins, healthy grains, and a variety of vegetables. They are designed to maintain overall health, energy levels, and wellness in adult dogs, ensuring that your furry friend gets everything they need from their daily meals.

Chapter Three

Golden Years: Recipes for Senior Dogs

Senior Chicken and Rice Comfort Stew

Ingredients:
- 1 lb boneless, skinless chicken thighs, diced
- 1 cup white rice, rinsed
- 1 cup chopped carrots
- 1/2 cup chopped zucchini
- 1/4 cup chopped parsley
- 4 cups low-sodium chicken broth

Instructions:
1. Place all ingredients in the slow cooker.
2. Stir to combine.
3. Cover and cook on low for 6-7 hours, until the chicken is tender and the rice is fully cooked.
4. Let it cool before serving.

Turkey and Sweet Potato Gentle Meal

Ingredients:
- 1 lb ground turkey
- 1 cup diced sweet potatoes
- 1/2 cup chopped green beans
- 1/2 cup chopped spinach
- 1/4 cup diced apples (core and seeds removed)
- 4 cups low-sodium chicken broth

Instructions:
1. Brown the ground turkey in a skillet over medium heat.
2. Transfer the turkey to the slow cooker.
3. Add the sweet potatoes, green beans, spinach, apples, and chicken broth.
4. Stir to combine and cover.
5. Cook on low for 6-8 hours, until the sweet potatoes are soft and the flavors are well-blended.
6. Allow the food to cool before serving.

Beef and Barley Senior Stew

Ingredients:
- 1 lb lean ground beef
- 1 cup barley
- 1 cup diced carrots
- 1/2 cup chopped peas
- 1/4 cup chopped parsley
- 4 cups low-sodium beef broth

Instructions:
1. Brown the ground beef in a skillet over medium heat.
2. Transfer the beef to the slow cooker.
3. Add the barley, carrots, peas, parsley, and beef broth.
4. Stir to combine and cover.
5. Cook on low for 7-8 hours, until the barley is tender and the beef is fully cooked.
6. Cool before serving.

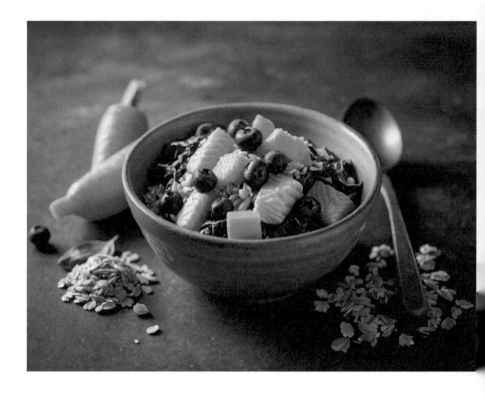

Salmon and Oatmeal Senior Special

Ingredients:
- 2 salmon fillets, skin removed, diced
- 1 cup rolled oats
- 1/2 cup chopped spinach
- 1/2 cup diced carrots
- 1/4 cup blueberries
- 4 cups water

Instructions:
1. Place all ingredients in the slow cooker.
2. Stir to combine.
3. Cover and cook on low for 5-6 hours, until the salmon is cooked and the oats are tender.
4. Let it cool before serving.

Lamb and Rice Senior Meal

Ingredients:
- 1 lb ground lamb
- 1 cup white rice, rinsed
- 1/2 cup chopped broccoli
- 1/2 cup diced carrots
- 1/4 cup chopped parsley
- 4 cups low-sodium chicken broth

Instructions:
1. Place all ingredients in the slow cooker.
2. Stir to combine.
3. Cover and cook on low for 6-7 hours, until the rice is tender and the lamb is fully cooked.
4. Cool before serving.

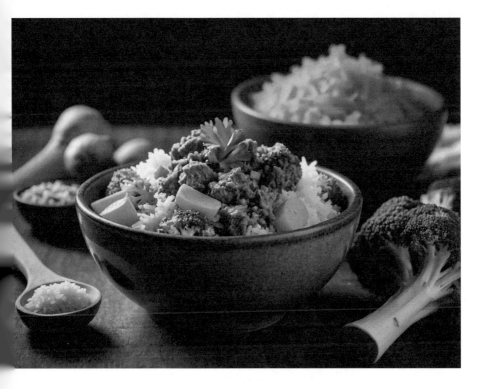

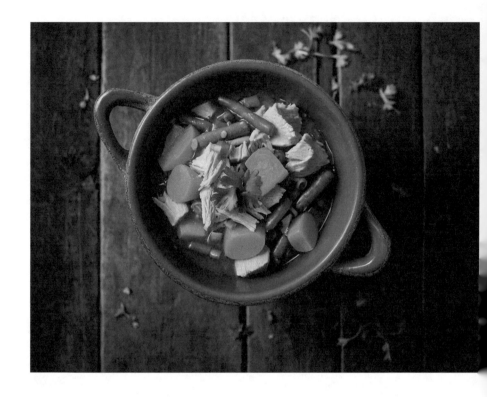

Chicken and Pumpkin Soft Stew

Ingredients:
- 1 lb boneless, skinless chicken breasts, diced
- 1 cup canned pumpkin (pure, unsweetened)
- 1/2 cup chopped green beans
- 1/2 cup chopped carrots
- 1/4 cup chopped parsley
- 4 cups low-sodium chicken broth

Instructions:
1. Place all ingredients in the slow cooker.
2. Stir to combine.
3. Cover and cook on low for 5-6 hours, until the chicken is fully cooked and th vegetables are tender.
4. Allow the food to cool before serving.

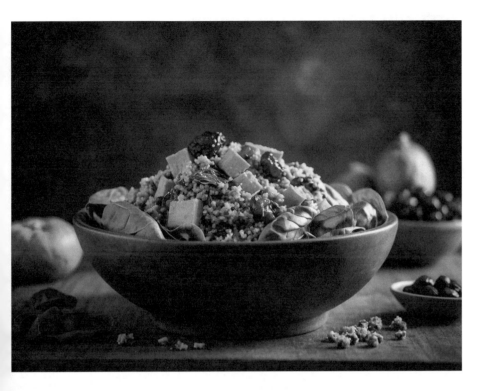

Turkey and Quinoa Gentle Stew

Ingredients:
- 1 lb ground turkey
- 1 cup quinoa, rinsed
- 1/2 cup diced sweet potatoes
- 1/2 cup chopped spinach
- 1/4 cup cranberries
- 4 cups low-sodium chicken broth

Instructions:
1. Brown the ground turkey in a skillet over medium heat.
2. Transfer the turkey to the slow cooker.
3. Add the quinoa, sweet potatoes, spinach, cranberries, and chicken broth.
4. Stir to combine.
5. Cover and cook on low for 6-7 hours, until the quinoa is tender and the turkey is fully cooked.
6. Let it cool before serving.

Beef and Potato Senior Delight

Ingredients:
- 1 lb lean ground beef
- 1 cup diced potatoes
- 1/2 cup chopped carrots
- 1/2 cup peas
- 1/4 cup chopped parsley
- 4 cups low-sodium beef broth

Instructions:
1. Brown the ground beef in a skillet over medium heat.
2. Transfer the beef to the slow cooker.
3. Add the potatoes, carrots, peas, parsley, and beef broth.
4. Stir to combine and cover.
5. Cook on low for 7-8 hours, until the potatoes are tender and the beef is fully cooked.
6. Cool before serving.

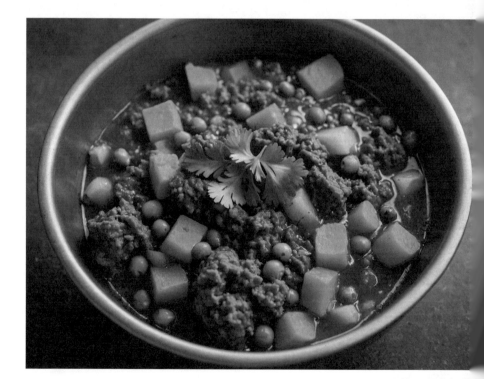

Chicken and Barley Senior Stew

Ingredients:
- 1 lb boneless, skinless chicken thighs, diced
- 1 cup barley
- 1/2 cup chopped zucchini
- 1/2 cup diced carrots
- 1/4 cup chopped parsley
- 4 cups low-sodium chicken broth

Instructions:
1. Place all ingredients in the slow cooker.
2. Stir to combine.
3. Cover and cook on low for 7-8 hours, until the barley is tender and the chicken is fully cooked.
4. Let it cool before serving.

Turkey and Lentil Senior Stew

Ingredients:
- 1 lb ground turkey
- 1 cup lentils, rinsed
- 1/2 cup chopped spinach
- 1/2 cup chopped carrots
- 1/4 cup chopped parsley
- 4 cups low-sodium chicken broth

Instructions:
1. Brown the ground turkey in a skillet over medium heat.
2. Transfer the turkey to the slow cooker.
3. Add the lentils, spinach, carrots, parsley, and chicken broth.
4. Stir to combine and cover.
5. Cook on low for 6-8 hours, until the lentils are tender and the turkey is fully cooked.
6. Cool before serving.

These recipes are designed to provide senior dogs with the nutrients they need while being gentle on their digestive systems. The ingredients are chosen to support joint health, provide easy digestion, and ensure that older dogs maintain a healthy weight and energy level.

Chapter Four

Special Diets: Allergy-Friendly and Grain-Free Recipes

Grain-Free Turkey and Sweet Potato Stew

Ingredients:
- 1 lb ground turkey
- 2 cups diced sweet potatoes
- 1/2 cup chopped green beans
- 1/2 cup chopped zucchini
- 1/4 cup cranberries
- 4 cups low-sodium chicken broth

Instructions:
1. Brown the ground turkey in a skillet over medium heat.
2. Transfer the turkey to the slow cooker.
3. Add the sweet potatoes, green beans, zucchini, cranberries, and chicken broth.
4. Stir to combine.
5. Cover and cook on low for 6-7 hours, until the sweet potatoes are tender and the turkey is fully cooked.
6. Let it cool before serving.

Duck and Pumpkin Grain-Free Delight

Ingredients:
- 1 lb ground duck
- 1 cup canned pumpkin (pure, unsweetened)
- 1/2 cup diced carrots
- 1/2 cup chopped spinach
- 1/4 cup blueberries
- 4 cups water

Instructions:
1. Place all ingredients in the slow cooker.
2. Stir to combine.
3. Cover and cook on low for 5-6 hours, until the duck is fully cooked and the vegetables are tender.
4. Allow the food to cool before serving.

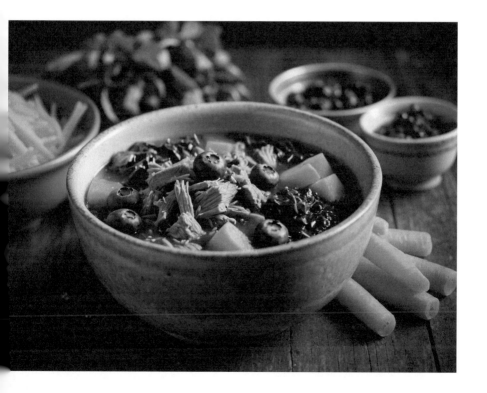

Salmon and Vegetable Grain-Free Feast

Ingredients:
- 2 salmon fillets, skin removed, diced
- 1 cup diced carrots
- 1/2 cup chopped green beans
- 1/2 cup chopped zucchini
- 1/4 cup chopped parsley
- 4 cups water

Instructions:
1. Place all ingredients in the slow cooker.
2. Stir to combine.
3. Cover and cook on low for 4-5 hours, until the salmon is cooked and the vegetables are tender.
4. Let it cool before serving.

Venison and Sweet Potato Grain-Free Meal

Ingredients:
- 1 lb ground venison
- 2 cups diced sweet potatoes
- 1/2 cup chopped green beans
- 1/2 cup chopped kale
- 1/4 cup chopped cranberries
- 4 cups water

Instructions:
1. Place all ingredients in the slow cooker.
2. Stir to combine.
3. Cover and cook on low for 6-8 hours, until the sweet potatoes are tender and the venison is fully cooked.
4. Let it cool before serving.

Lamb and Butternut Squash Stew

Ingredients:
- 1 lb ground lamb
- 2 cups diced butternut squash
- 1/2 cup chopped spinach
- 1/2 cup chopped carrots
- 1/4 cup chopped apples (core and seeds removed)
- 4 cups low-sodium chicken broth

Instructions:
1. Place all ingredients in the slow cooker.
2. Stir to combine.
3. Cover and cook on low for 6-7 hours, until the squash is tender and the lamb is fully cooked.
4. Cool before serving.

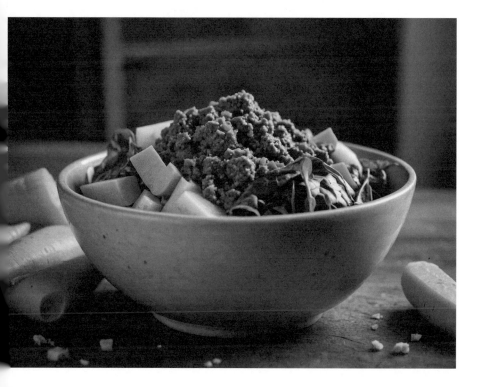

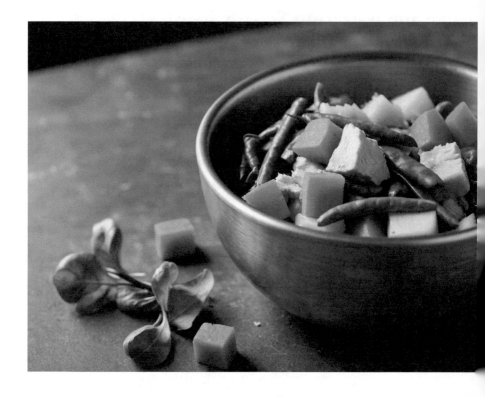

Chicken and Green Bean Grain-Free Dinner

Ingredients:
- 1 lb boneless, skinless chicken thighs, diced
- 1 cup chopped green beans
- 1/2 cup diced carrots
- 1/2 cup chopped spinach
- 1/4 cup diced apples (core and seeds removed)
- 4 cups low-sodium chicken broth

Instructions:
1. Place all ingredients in the slow cooker.
2. Stir to combine.
3. Cover and cook on low for 6-7 hours, until the chicken is tender and the vegetable are cooked through.
4. Cool before serving.

Beef and Pumpkin Grain-Free Stew

Ingredients:
- 1 lb lean ground beef
- 1 cup canned pumpkin (pure, unsweetened)
- 1/2 cup chopped zucchini
- 1/2 cup chopped carrots
- 1/4 cup chopped parsley
- 4 cups low-sodium beef broth

Instructions:
1. Brown the ground beef in a skillet over medium heat.
2. Transfer the beef to the slow cooker.
3. Add the pumpkin, zucchini, carrots, parsley, and beef broth.
4. Stir to combine and cover.
5. Cook on low for 5-6 hours, until the vegetables are tender and the flavors are well-blended.
6. Cool before serving.

Turkey and Green Bean Grain-Free Stew

Ingredients:
- 1 lb ground turkey
- 1 cup chopped green beans
- 1/2 cup diced sweet potatoes
- 1/2 cup chopped kale
- 1/4 cup chopped apples (core and seeds removed)
- 4 cups low-sodium chicken broth

Instructions:
1. Brown the ground turkey in a skillet over medium heat.
2. Transfer the turkey to the slow cooker.
3. Add the green beans, sweet potatoes, kale, apples, and chicken broth.
4. Stir to combine.
5. Cover and cook on low for 6-7 hours, until the sweet potatoes are tender and the turkey is fully cooked.
6. Let it cool before serving.

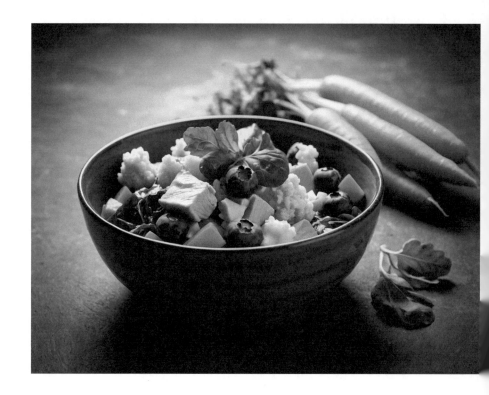

Chicken and Cauliflower Grain-Free Meal

Ingredients:
- 1 lb boneless, skinless chicken breasts, diced
- 1 cup chopped cauliflower
- 1/2 cup diced carrots
- 1/2 cup chopped spinach
- 1/4 cup blueberries
- 4 cups water

Instructions:
1. Place all ingredients in the slow cooker.
2. Stir to combine.
3. Cover and cook on low for 5-6 hours, until the chicken is fully cooked and the vegetables are tender.
4. Allow the food to cool before serving.

Pork and Apple Grain-Free Stew

Ingredients:
- 1 lb ground pork
- 1 cup diced apples (core and seeds removed)
- 1/2 cup chopped carrots
- 1/2 cup chopped kale
- 1/4 cup cranberries
- 4 cups low-sodium chicken broth

Instructions:
1. Place all ingredients in the slow cooker.
2. Stir to combine.
3. Cover and cook on low for 6-7 hours, until the pork is fully cooked and the apples and vegetables are tender.
4. Cool before serving.

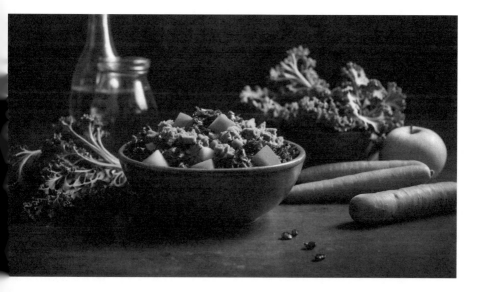

These grain-free and allergy-friendly recipes are designed for dogs with food sensitivities or allergies. They focus on high-quality proteins and a variety of vegetables, enuring that your dog gets all the essential nutrients while avoiding common allergens ike grains and gluten.

Chapter Five

Weight Management: Low-Calorie Recipes

Lean Turkey and Veggie Slim-Down Stew

Ingredients:
- 1 lb ground turkey (extra lean)
- 1 cup diced zucchini
- 1/2 cup diced carrots
- 1/2 cup chopped green beans
- 1/4 cup chopped spinach
- 4 cups low-sodium chicken broth

Instructions:
1. Brown the ground turkey in a skillet over medium heat.
2. Transfer the turkey to the slow cooker.
3. Add the zucchini, carrots, green beans, spinach, and chicken broth.
4. Stir to combine and cover.
5. Cook on low for 6-7 hours, until the vegetables are tender and the turkey is fully cooked.
6. Let it cool before serving.

Chicken and Cauliflower Slim-Meal

Ingredients:
- 1 lb boneless, skinless chicken breasts, diced
- 1 cup chopped cauliflower
- 1/2 cup chopped kale
- 1/2 cup diced carrots
- 4 cups water

Instructions:
1. Place all ingredients in the slow cooker.
2. Stir to combine.
3. Cover and cook on low for 5-6 hours, until the chicken is fully cooked and the vegetables are tender.
4. Allow the food to cool before serving.

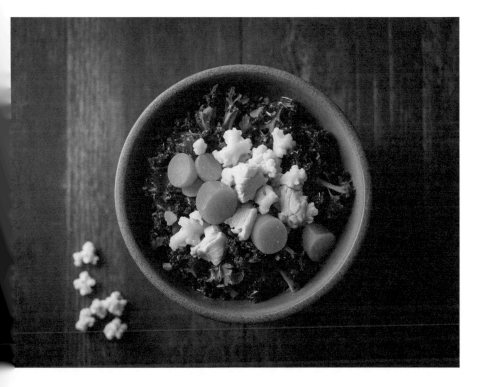

Low-Cal Beef and Veggie Medley

Ingredients:
- 1 lb lean ground beef
- 1 cup diced celery
- 1/2 cup chopped spinach
- 1/2 cup chopped green beans
- 1/4 cup diced apples (core and seeds removed)
- 4 cups low-sodium beef broth

Instructions:
1. Brown the ground beef in a skillet over medium heat.
2. Transfer the beef to the slow cooker.
3. Add the celery, spinach, green beans, apples, and beef broth.
4. Stir to combine and cover.
5. Cook on low for 6-7 hours, until the vegetables are tender and the beef is fully cooked.
6. Cool before serving.

Salmon and Green Bean Low-Calorie Feast

Ingredients:
- 2 salmon fillets, skin removed, diced
- 1 cup chopped green beans
- 1/2 cup diced zucchini
- 1/4 cup chopped carrots
- 4 cups water

Instructions:
1. Place all ingredients in the slow cooker.
2. Stir to combine.
3. Cover and cook on low for 4-5 hours, until the salmon is cooked and the vegetables are tender.
4. Let it cool before serving.

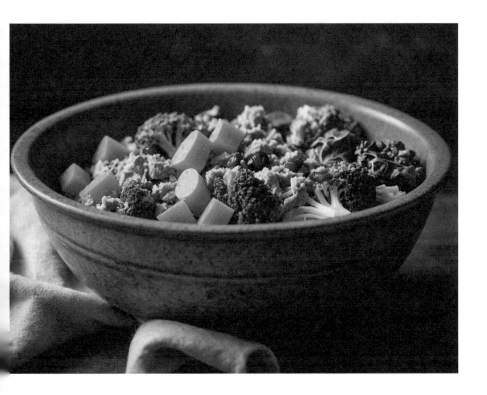

Turkey and Broccoli Light Meal

Ingredients:
- 1 lb ground turkey (extra lean)
- 1 cup chopped broccoli
- 1/2 cup chopped spinach
- 1/2 cup diced carrots
- 1/4 cup cranberries
- 4 cups low-sodium chicken broth

Instructions:
1. Brown the ground turkey in a skillet over medium heat.
2. Transfer the turkey to the slow cooker.
3. Add the broccoli, spinach, carrots, cranberries, and chicken broth.
4. Stir to combine and cover.
5. Cook on low for 6-7 hours, until the vegetables are tender and the turkey is fully cooked.
6. Cool before serving.

Chicken and Pumpkin Slim Stew

Ingredients:
- 1 lb boneless, skinless chicken thighs, diced
- 1 cup canned pumpkin (pure, unsweetened)
- 1/2 cup chopped green beans
- 1/2 cup chopped spinach
- 1/4 cup chopped parsley
- 4 cups low-sodium chicken broth

Instructions:
1. Place all ingredients in the slow cooker.
2. Stir to combine.
3. Cover and cook on low for 5-6 hours, until the chicken is fully cooked and the vegetables are tender.
4. Allow the food to cool before serving.

Low-Cal Lamb and Veggie Dinner

Ingredients:
- 1 lb ground lamb (extra lean)
- 1 cup chopped zucchini
- 1/2 cup chopped spinach
- 1/2 cup diced carrots
- 1/4 cup diced apples (core and seeds removed)
- 4 cups low-sodium chicken broth

Instructions:
1. Brown the ground lamb in a skillet over medium heat.
2. Transfer the lamb to the slow cooker.
3. Add the zucchini, spinach, carrots, apples, and chicken broth.
4. Stir to combine and cover.
5. Cook on low for 6-7 hours, until the vegetables are tender and the lamb is full cooked.
6. Cool before serving.

White Fish and Veggie Low-Calorie Stew

Ingredients:
- 2 white fish fillets (such as cod or tilapia), skin removed, diced
- 1 cup chopped green beans
- 1/2 cup diced zucchini
- 1/2 cup chopped spinach
- 4 cups water

Instructions:
1. Place all ingredients in the slow cooker.
2. Stir to combine.
3. Cover and cook on low for 4-5 hours, until the fish is cooked and the vegetables are tender.
4. Let it cool before serving.

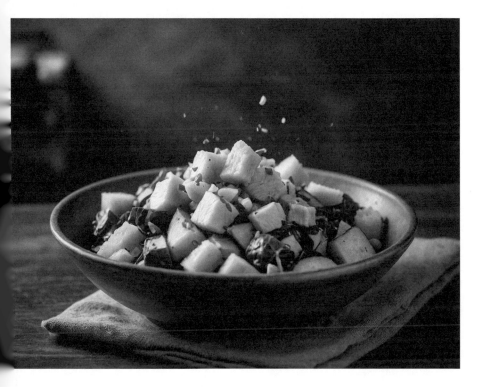

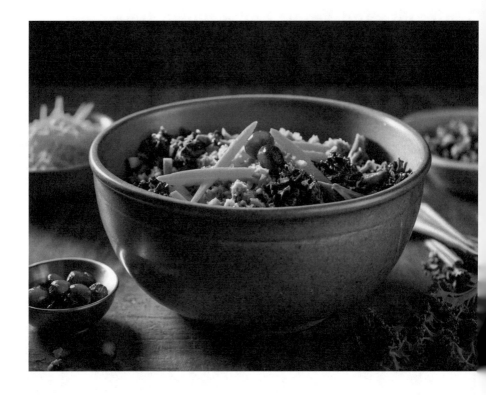

Turkey and Green Bean Light Feast

Ingredients:
- 1 lb ground turkey (extra lean)
- 1 cup chopped green beans
- 1/2 cup diced carrots
- 1/2 cup chopped kale
- 1/4 cup cranberries
- 4 cups low-sodium chicken broth

Instructions:
1. Brown the ground turkey in a skillet over medium heat.
2. Transfer the turkey to the slow cooker.
3. Add the green beans, carrots, kale, cranberries, and chicken broth.
4. Stir to combine.
5. Cover and cook on low for 6-7 hours, until the vegetables are tender and the turkey is fully cooked.
6. Cool before serving.

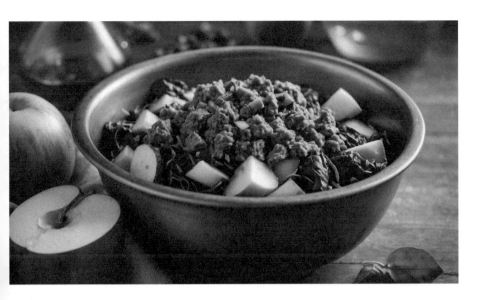

Pork and Apple Slimming Stew

Ingredients:
- 1 lb ground pork (lean)
- 1 cup diced apples (core and seeds removed)
- 1/2 cup chopped zucchini
- 1/2 cup chopped spinach
- 4 cups low-sodium chicken broth

Instructions:
1. Place all ingredients in the slow cooker.
2. Stir to combine.
3. Cover and cook on low for 5-6 hours, until the pork is fully cooked and the vegetables are tender.
4. Allow the food to cool before serving.

These low-calorie recipes are designed to help manage your dog's weight while providing essential nutrients. They focus on lean proteins, low-calorie vegetables, and simple flavors to keep your dog satisfied without unnecessary calories.

Chapter Six

Healing and Recovery: Recipes for Dogs with Health Issues

Gentle Chicken and Rice Recovery Stew

For dogs with upset stomachs or sensitive digestion.

Ingredients:
- 1 lb boneless, skinless chicken breasts, diced
- 1 cup white rice, rinsed
- 1/2 cup diced carrots
- 1/2 cup chopped green beans
- 4 cups low-sodium chicken broth

Instructions:
1. Place all ingredients in the slow cooker.
2. Stir to combine.
3. Cover and cook on low for 6-7 hours, until the chicken is fully cooked and the rice is tender.
4. Allow the food to cool before serving.

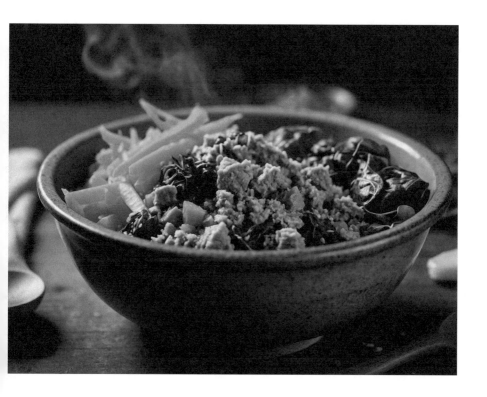

Soothing Turkey and Pumpkin Stew

For dogs with digestive issues or recovering from illness.

Ingredients:
- 1 lb ground turkey
- 1 cup canned pumpkin (pure, unsweetened)
- 1/2 cup diced carrots
- 1/2 cup chopped spinach
- 4 cups water

Instructions:
1. Brown the ground turkey in a skillet over medium heat.
2. Transfer the turkey to the slow cooker.
3. Add the pumpkin, carrots, spinach, and water.
4. Stir to combine.
5. Cover and cook on low for 5-6 hours, until the turkey is fully cooked and the vegetables are tender.
6. Let it cool before serving.

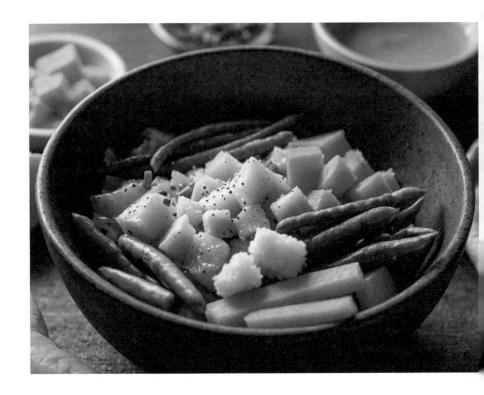

Healing Fish and Sweet Potato Stew

For dogs with skin and coat issues.

Ingredients:
- 2 white fish fillets (such as cod or tilapia), skin removed, diced
- 1 cup diced sweet potatoes
- 1/2 cup chopped green beans
- 1/2 cup chopped carrots
- 4 cups water

Instructions:
1. Place all ingredients in the slow cooker.
2. Stir to combine.
3. Cover and cook on low for 4-5 hours, until the fish is cooked and the vegetables are tender.
4. Let it cool before serving.

Kidney Support Beef and Rice Stew

For dogs with kidney issues.

Ingredients:
- 1 lb lean ground beef
- 1 cup white rice, rinsed
- 1/2 cup chopped zucchini
- 1/2 cup diced carrots
- 4 cups water

Instructions:
1. Brown the ground beef in a skillet over medium heat.
2. Transfer the beef to the slow cooker.
3. Add the rice, zucchini, carrots, and water.
4. Stir to combine.
5. Cover and cook on low for 6-7 hours, until the rice is tender and the beef is fully cooked.
6. Cool before serving.

Liver Support Turkey and Sweet Potato Stew

For dogs with liver issues.

Ingredients:
- 1 lb ground turkey
- 1 cup diced sweet potatoes
- 1/2 cup chopped green beans
- 1/2 cup chopped spinach
- 4 cups water

Instructions:
1. Brown the ground turkey in a skillet over medium heat.
2. Transfer the turkey to the slow cooker.
3. Add the sweet potatoes, green beans, spinach, and water.
4. Stir to combine.
5. Cover and cook on low for 6-7 hours, until the sweet potatoes are tender and the turkey is fully cooked.
6. Let it cool before serving.

Anti-Inflammatory Chicken and Oats Stew

For dogs with joint pain or arthritis.

Ingredients:
- 1 lb boneless, skinless chicken thighs, diced
- 1 cup rolled oats
- 1/2 cup chopped spinach
- 1/2 cup diced carrots
- 1/4 cup blueberries
- 4 cups low-sodium chicken broth

Instructions:
1. Place all ingredients in the slow cooker.
2. Stir to combine.
3. Cover and cook on low for 6-7 hours, until the oats are tender and the chicken is fully cooked.
4. Cool before serving.

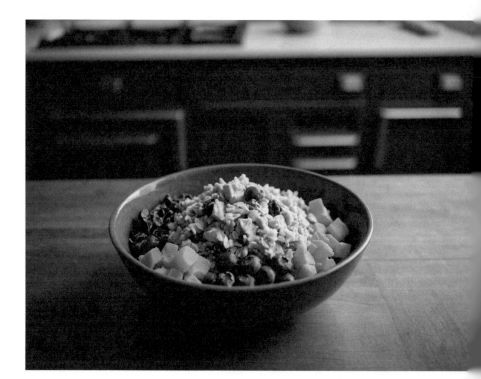

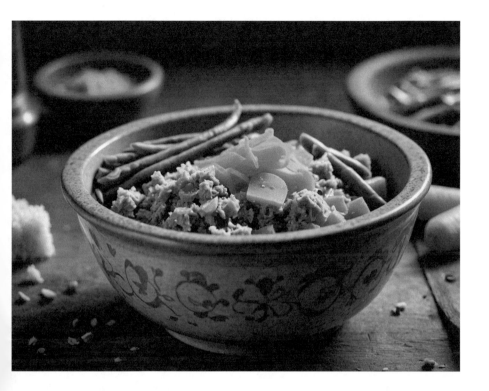

Low-Fat Turkey and Carrot Stew

For dogs recovering from pancreatitis.

Ingredients:
- 1 lb ground turkey (extra lean)
- 1 cup diced carrots
- 1/2 cup chopped green beans
- 4 cups water

Instructions:
1. Brown the ground turkey in a skillet over medium heat.
2. Transfer the turkey to the slow cooker.
3. Add the carrots, green beans, and water.
4. Stir to combine.
5. Cover and cook on low for 5-6 hours, until the turkey is fully cooked and the vegetables are tender.
6. Let it cool before serving.

Digestive Support Lamb and Rice Stew

For dogs with digestive issues or food sensitivities.

Ingredients:
- 1 lb ground lamb
- 1 cup white rice, rinsed
- 1/2 cup diced zucchini
- 1/2 cup chopped carrots
- 4 cups water

Instructions:
1. Place all ingredients in the slow cooker.
2. Stir to combine.
3. Cover and cook on low for 6-7 hours, until the rice is tender and the lamb is fully cooked.
4. Cool before serving.

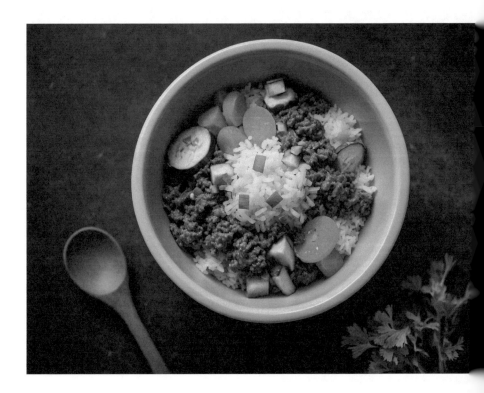

Liver Detox Chicken and Apple Stew

For dogs in need of a liver detox.

Ingredients:
- 1 lb boneless, skinless chicken breasts, diced
- 1 cup diced apples (core and seeds removed)
- 1/2 cup chopped kale
- 1/2 cup diced carrots
- 4 cups low-sodium chicken broth

Instructions:
1. Place all ingredients in the slow cooker.
2. Stir to combine.
3. Cover and cook on low for 6-7 hours, until the chicken is fully cooked and the vegetables are tender.
4. Let it cool before serving.

Weight Gain Support Beef and Sweet Potato Stew

For dogs recovering from illness and needing to gain weight.

Ingredients:
- 1 lb lean ground beef
- 1 cup diced sweet potatoes
- 1/2 cup chopped peas
- 1/2 cup diced carrots
- 4 cups low-sodium beef broth

Instructions:
1. Brown the ground beef in a skillet over medium heat.
2. Transfer the beef to the slow cooker.
3. Add the sweet potatoes, peas, carrots, and beef broth.
4. Stir to combine and cover.
5. Cook on low for 6-7 hours, until the sweet potatoes are tender and the beef is fully cooked.
6. Cool before serving.

These recipes are tailored to meet the specific needs of dogs dealing with various health issues. They focus on gentle ingredients that support recovery and promote overall well-being, while still being delicious and satisfying for your dog.

Chapter Seven

Treats and Snacks: Healthy Slow Cooker Snacks

Peanut Butter and Banana Bites

Ingredients:
- 1 cup rolled oats
- 1/2 cup natural peanut butter (xylitol-free)
- 1/2 cup mashed ripe bananas
- 1/4 cup chopped apples (core and seeds removed)
- 1/4 cup water

Instructions:
1. Combine all ingredients in the slow cooker.
2. Stir to mix well.
3. Form small bite-sized balls or drop spoonfuls into the slow cooker.
4. Cook on low for 2-3 hours until firm.
5. Allow to cool completely before serving.

Chicken and Sweet Potato Chews

Ingredients:
- 1 lb boneless, skinless chicken breasts, sliced thin
- 1 large sweet potato, peeled and sliced into thin rounds

Instructions:
1. Layer the chicken slices and sweet potato rounds in the slow cooker.
2. Cover and cook on low for 4-6 hours until both are dehydrated and chewy.
3. Let the chews cool completely before serving.

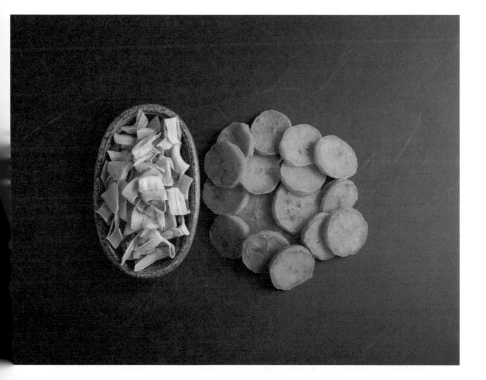

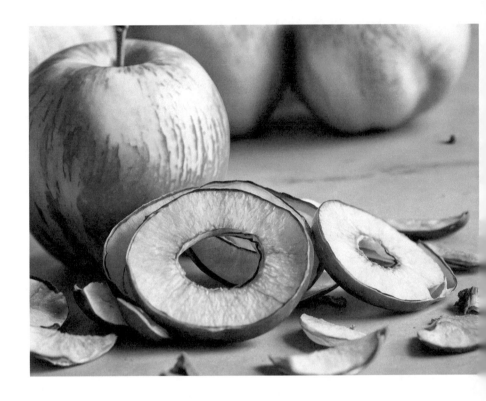

Apple and Cinnamon Dog Chips

Ingredients:
- 2 large apples (core and seeds removed), sliced thin
- 1 tsp cinnamon (optional)

Instructions:
1. Place the apple slices in the slow cooker in a single layer.
2. Sprinkle with cinnamon if desired.
3. Cover and cook on low for 4-6 hours until the apples are dehydrated and crispy.
4. Let the chips cool completely before serving.

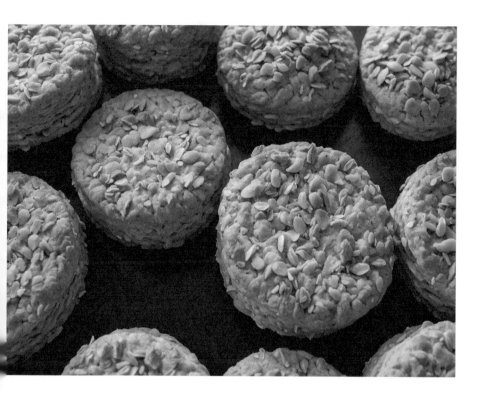

Pumpkin and Oatmeal Biscuits

Ingredients:
- 1 cup canned pumpkin (pure, unsweetened)
- 1 cup rolled oats
- 1/4 cup applesauce (unsweetened)
- 1/4 cup water

Instructions:
1. Combine all ingredients in the slow cooker and mix well.
2. Form small biscuits or drop spoonfuls into the slow cooker.
3. Cook on low for 3-4 hours until the biscuits are firm.
4. Allow to cool completely before serving.

Carrot and Apple Dog Treats

Ingredients:
- 1 cup grated carrots
- 1/2 cup rolled oats
- 1/4 cup natural peanut butter (xylitol-free)
- 1/4 cup chopped apples (core and seeds removed)

Instructions:
1. Mix all ingredients together in the slow cooker.
2. Form small treats or drop spoonfuls into the slow cooker.
3. Cook on low for 3-4 hours until the treats are firm.
4. Let the treats cool completely before serving.

Salmon and Sweet Potato Dog Jerky

Ingredients:
- 2 salmon fillets, skin removed, sliced thin
- 1 large sweet potato, peeled and sliced thin

Instructions:
1. Place the salmon slices and sweet potato slices in the slow cooker.
2. Cover and cook on low for 4-6 hours until dehydrated and chewy.
3. Let the jerky cool completely before serving.

Banana and Coconut Dog Bites

Ingredients:
- 1 cup mashed ripe bananas
- 1/2 cup rolled oats
- 1/4 cup unsweetened shredded coconut
- 1/4 cup natural peanut butter (xylitol-free)

Instructions:
1. Mix all ingredients together in the slow cooker.
2. Form small bite-sized balls or drop spoonfuls into the slow cooker.
3. Cook on low for 2-3 hours until firm.
4. Let the bites cool completely before serving.

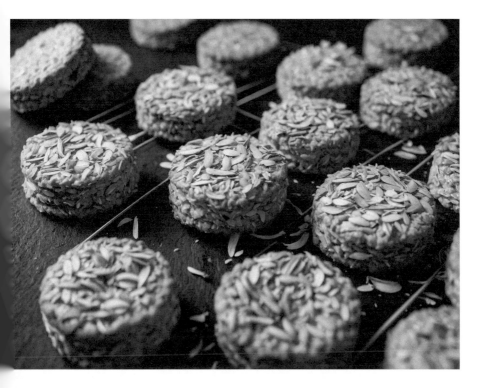

Beef and Carrot Crunchies

Ingredients:
- 1 lb lean ground beef
- 1 cup grated carrots
- 1/4 cup rolled oats

Instructions:
1. Brown the ground beef in a skillet over medium heat and drain excess fat.
2. Combine the cooked beef, grated carrots, and oats in the slow cooker.
3. Form small treat-sized balls or patties.
4. Cook on low for 3-4 hours until firm.
5. Allow to cool completely before serving.

Blueberry and Yogurt Dog Treats

Ingredients:
- 1 cup rolled oats
- 1/2 cup plain Greek yogurt (unsweetened)
- 1/2 cup fresh blueberries
- 1/4 cup water

Instructions:
1. Combine all ingredients in the slow cooker and mix well.
2. Form small treats or drop spoonfuls into the slow cooker.
3. Cook on low for 2-3 hours until firm.
4. Let the treats cool completely before serving.

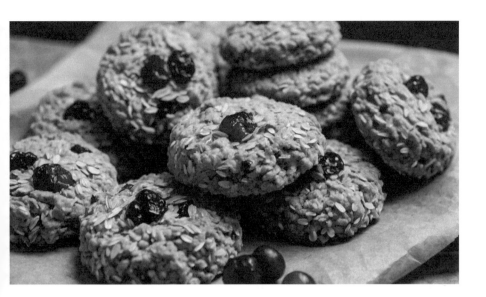

Turkey and Cranberry Dog Biscuits

Ingredients:
- 1 lb ground turkey
- 1/2 cup cranberries (unsweetened)
- 1/2 cup rolled oats
- 1/4 cup applesauce (unsweetened)

Instructions:
1. Brown the ground turkey in a skillet over medium heat and drain excess fat.
2. Combine the cooked turkey, cranberries, oats, and applesauce in the slow cooker.
3. Form small biscuits or patties.
4. Cook on low for 3-4 hours until firm.
5. Let the biscuits cool completely before serving.

These healthy slow cooker treats and snacks are designed to be nutritious and tasty, perfect for rewarding your dog or providing a small snack between meals. Each recipe focuses on wholesome ingredients that are easy on your dog's digestive system while still being enjoyable for them to eat.

Ingredient Substitutions and Customization

One of the benefits of making homemade dog food is the ability to customize meals to suit your dog's individual needs and preferences. This section will guide you through various ingredient substitutions and customization tips to ensure that each recipe is tailored specifically for your dog. Whether you're dealing with food allergies, dietary restrictions, or just a picky eater, these tips will help you create meals that your dog will love while maintaining the nutritional balance they need.

Common Ingredient Substitutions

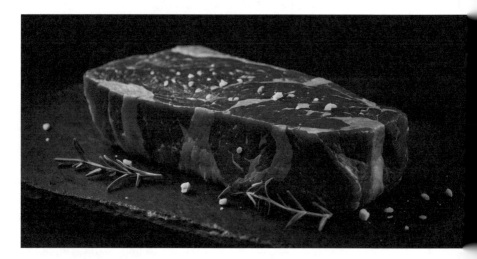

1. Protein Sources:

   o Chicken: If your dog is allergic to chicken, you can substitute it with turkey, lean beef, lamb, or fish (like salmon or white fish). Always ensure that the protein source is lean to avoid unnecessary fat.

○ Turkey: Substitute with chicken, lean ground beef, or duck. For a more exotic option, venison can also be used if available.

○ Beef: If your dog has a sensitivity to beef, substitute with turkey, chicken, lamb, or pork. For a more novel protein, you can use rabbit or bison.

○ Fish: Salmon and white fish are commonly used, but if your dog prefers a different flavor, you can substitute with cod, tilapia, or even sardines (just ensure they are boneless and low in sodium).

2. Grains:

○ Rice (White or Brown): If your dog is sensitive to grains, you can use grain-free alternatives like quinoa or barley, or skip grains altogether and focus on starchy vegetables like sweet potatoes or butternut squash.

○ Oats: If your dog has an issue with oats, consider using quinoa or millet as a substitute. Both are gluten-free and provide a similar texture and nutritional profile.

○ Barley: This can be substituted with brown rice, quinoa, or even buckwheat, which is gluten-free and rich in fiber.

3. Vegetables:

○ Carrots: If your dog doesn't like carrots or is allergic, you can substitute with other root vegetables like parsnips or turnips. Zucchini and butternut squash are also great alternatives.

○ Green Beans: Substitute with peas, spinach, or kale. These greens provide similar vitamins and minerals, ensuring your dog's meal remains balanced.

○ Sweet Potatoes: For dogs that don't tolerate sweet potatoes well, you can use regular potatoes, butternut squash, or pumpkin. Each provides a good source of fiber and vitamins.

4. Fruits:

○ Apples: If your dog doesn't enjoy apples or has a sensitivity, pears make an excellent substitute. Both are low in calories and high in fiber.

○ Blueberries: Substitute with other berries like strawberries, raspberries, or blackberries. All are rich in antioxidants and safe for dogs in moderation.

○ Cranberries: If cranberries are not available, you can use chopped dried apricots (unsweetened and free of preservatives) or even diced pears.

Customizing for Dietary Needs

1. Allergies and Sensitivities:

- If your dog has food allergies or sensitivities, it's crucial to identify the offending ingredients and remove them from the diet. The recipes provided offer flexibility with protein and vegetable choices, so you can easily make substitutions.

- For dogs with multiple food sensitivities, consider using novel proteins like rabbit, venison, or duck, which are less likely to cause an allergic reaction.

- Grain-free recipes are provided for dogs with grain sensitivities. If you need to further customize, focus on using starchy vegetables like sweet potatoes, pumpkin, and squash as carbohydrate sources.

2. Weight Management:

- If your dog needs to lose weight, focus on lean proteins like chicken breast, turkey, and white fish. Avoid fatty cuts of meat and limit the use of high-calorie ingredients like sweet potatoes and pumpkin.

- Increase the proportion of low-calorie vegetables like zucchini, green beans, and spinach. These can help your dog feel full without adding extra calories.

- Portion control is key in weight management. Use a kitchen scale to measure portions accurately and ensure that your dog is getting the right amount of food for their size and activity level.

3. Digestive Issues:

- For dogs with sensitive stomachs or digestive issues, stick to simple, easily digestible ingredients. Chicken and rice or turkey and sweet potatoes are classic combinations that are gentle on the stomach.

- Avoid ingredients that are known to cause gas or bloating, such as broccoli, cabbage, and beans. Instead, use carrots, zucchini, and spinach which are easier to digest.

- Incorporating a small amount of plain, unsweetened yogurt or probiotic into your dog's diet can help support healthy digestion.

4. Picky Eaters:

- If your dog is a picky eater, you may need to experiment with different flavors and textures. Some dogs prefer moist, stew-like meals, while other enjoy a bit more crunch.

○ Adding a small amount of low-sodium chicken or beef broth to meals can enhance flavor and encourage eating.

○ For dogs that enjoy a bit of sweetness, incorporating fruits like apples or blueberries into their meals can make the food more appealing.

Customizing Portion Sizes

Every dog is unique, and portion sizes should be customized based on your dog's age, weight, activity level, and overall health. Here's a general guideline to help you determine the appropriate portion size:

- Puppies: Require more frequent, smaller meals throughout the day. Typically, they eat 3-4 meals per day.

- Adult Dogs: Usually eat 2 meals per day, but portion sizes will vary depending on their size and activity level. Active dogs may need larger portions or additional snacks.

- Senior Dogs: Often require smaller, more frequent meals due to slower metabolism and reduced activity levels.

To customize portions:

1. Use a Kitchen Scale: Weigh your dog's food to ensure accurate portion sizes. This is especially important for weight management and dogs with specific dietary needs.

2. Monitor Body Condition: Regularly assess your dog's body condition and adjust portion sizes accordingly. If your dog is gaining or losing weight, adjust the portions to maintain a healthy weight.

3. Consult Your Vet: If you're unsure about the right portion size for your dog, consult your veterinarian. They can provide guidance based on your dog's specific needs.

Rotating Ingredients

Variety is essential for a balanced diet, and rotating ingredients can help ensure that your dog gets a broad spectrum of nutrients. Here's how to effectively rotate ingredients:

- Protein Rotation: Rotate between different protein sources like chicken, turkey, beef, and fish. This prevents your dog from developing a sensitivity to any one protein and ensures a variety of amino acids.

- Vegetable Rotation: Include a mix of vegetables in your dog's meals, rotating between carrots, zucchini, green beans, spinach, and sweet potatoes. This provides a range of vitamins and minerals.

• Fruit Rotation: Occasionally include fruits like apples, blueberries, and cranberries in your dog's diet for antioxidants and fiber. Rotate these to prevent boredom and maintain interest in meals.

This section empowers you to customize the recipes to meet your dog's specific needs, ensuring that each meal is as beneficial and enjoyable as possible. Whether your dog has allergies, weight concerns, or is simply a picky eater, these tips and substitutions will help you craft the perfect meal every time.

Supplements and Add-Ins

While the recipes in this book are designed to provide a balanced diet for your dog, there are times when adding specific supplements or enhancing meals with extra nutrients can be beneficial. This section will guide you through various supplements and add-ins that can help boost your dog's overall health, address specific health concerns, or simply add some extra flavor and variety to their meals.

Common Supplements for Dogs

1. Fish Oil (Omega-3 Fatty Acids):

   o Benefits: Omega-3 fatty acids found in fish oil are excellent for promoting a healthy coat and skin, reducing inflammation, supporting heart health, and improving cognitive function in older dogs.

   o How to Use: Add a few drops of fish oil directly to your dog's meal just before serving. Be sure to follow the recommended dosage based on your dog's size and weight. Always consult with your vet before introducing fish oil, especially if your dog has a history of pancreatitis or other fat-sensitive conditions.

2. Glucosamine and Chondroitin:

   o Benefits: These supplements are often used to support joint health, especially in older dogs or those with arthritis. They help maintain healthy cartilage and alleviate joint pain and stiffness.

   o How to Use: Glucosamine and chondroitin are usually available in tablet, powder, or liquid form. Mix the appropriate dosage into your dog's food based on their weight. These supplements are most effective when used consistently over time.

3. Probiotics:

   o Benefits: Probiotics promote healthy digestion by maintaining a balanced gut microbiome. They can help with issues like diarrhea, constipation, and bloating, and support overall digestive health.

- How to Use: Probiotics are available in powder, capsule, or chewable forms. Simply sprinkle the recommended amount over your dog's food or mix it in thoroughly. Yogurt can also be a natural source of probiotics, but ensure it's plain and unsweetened.

4. Digestive Enzymes:

- Benefits: Digestive enzymes help your dog break down food more efficiently, aiding in nutrient absorption and reducing digestive discomfort. This can be especially helpful for dogs with pancreatic insufficiency or those who struggle with digesting certain foods.

- How to Use: Digestive enzyme supplements are typically added directly to your dog's food at mealtime. Follow the dosage instructions on the product packaging or consult with your veterinarian for guidance.

5. Multivitamins:

- Benefits: A high-quality multivitamin can help fill in any nutritional gaps in your dog's diet, providing essential vitamins and minerals that support overall health, including immune function, bone health, and energy levels.

- How to Use: Multivitamins are available in various forms, including chewable tablets, powders, and liquids. Choose one that is appropriate for your dog's size and age, and mix it into their food as directed.

6. Coconut Oil:

- Benefits: Coconut oil is rich in medium-chain triglycerides (MCTs) which can provide a quick source of energy and support skin and coat health. It also has anti-inflammatory and anti-bacterial properties.

- How to Use: Add a small amount (about 1 teaspoon for small dogs, 1 tablespoon for large dogs) to your dog's food. Start with a smaller amount and gradually increase as tolerated.

7. Turmeric:

- Benefits: Turmeric is a natural anti-inflammatory that can help alleviate joint pain and support overall health. It also has antioxidant properties and can aid in digestion.

- How to Use: Mix a small amount of turmeric powder (about 1/8 teaspoon for small dogs, up to 1/2 teaspoon for large dogs) into your dog's meal. You can also create a "golden paste" by mixing turmeric with a bit of coconut oil and black pepper to enhance absorption.

8. Pumpkin:

- Benefits: Pumpkin is an excellent source of fiber and can help regulate your dog's digestion, making it useful for both diarrhea and constipation. It's also rich in vitamins A and C.

- How to Use: Add a tablespoon or two of canned pumpkin (pure, unsweetened) to your dog's meal. Avoid pumpkin pie filling, which contains added sugars and spices that aren't safe for dogs.

9. Bone Broth:

- Benefits: Bone broth is rich in nutrients like collagen, glycine, and glucosamine, which support joint health, gut health, and overall hydration. It's also highly palatable, making it a great add-in for picky eaters.

- How to Use: Pour a small amount of bone broth over your dog's food or mix it into their meal. Be sure to use a bone broth made specifically for pets or make your own without added salt, onions, or garlic.

10. Flaxseed:

- Benefits: Flaxseed is a great source of omega-3 fatty acids and fiber, supporting skin and coat health as well as digestion. It's also a good plant-based alternative to fish oil.

- How to Use: Ground flaxseed can be sprinkled over your dog's food (about 1/2 teaspoon for small dogs, up to 2 teaspoons for large dogs). Make sure to store ground flaxseed in the refrigerator to keep it fresh.

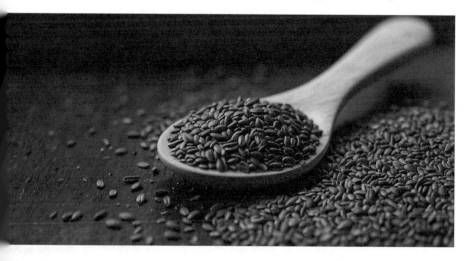

Adding Supplements to Recipes

When incorporating supplements into your dog's homemade meals, it's important to remember a few key points:

1. Start Slowly: Introduce supplements one at a time and in small amounts to ensure your dog tolerates them well. Watch for any adverse reactions, such as gastrointestinal upset or changes in behavior.

2. Follow Dosage Instructions: More is not always better when it comes to supplements. Always follow the dosage recommendations based on your dog's weight and consult your veterinarian if you're unsure.

3. Mix Thoroughly: To ensure that your dog receives the full benefit of the supplements, mix them thoroughly into the food so that every bite is balanced and nutritious.

4. Consider Your Dog's Specific Needs: Not all dogs require the same supplements. Consider your dog's age, health condition, and specific dietary needs when choosing which supplements to include.

5. Consult with Your Veterinarian: Before adding new supplements to your dog's diet, it's always a good idea to consult with your veterinarian. They can provide guidance on the most appropriate supplements and ensure there are no contraindications with any medications your dog may be taking.

Enhancing Flavor with Add-Ins

In addition to supplements, you can also use various add-ins to enhance the flavor and nutritional value of your dog's meals. These add-ins can be especially helpful if your dog is a picky eater or if you want to add variety to their diet.

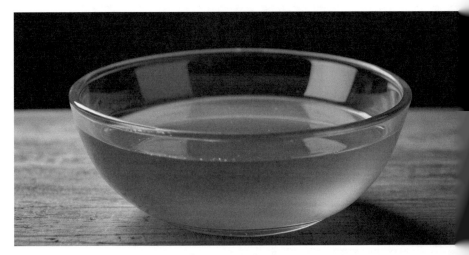

1. Low-Sodium Broth: Adding a small amount of low-sodium chicken or beef broth to your dog's meal can make it more flavorful and appealing. It's also a great way to increase your dog's fluid intake.

2. Cottage Cheese: A small spoonful of low-fat cottage cheese can add extra

protein and calcium to your dog's meal. It's also a tasty treat for dogs who enjoy dairy.

3. Plain Yogurt: Plain, unsweetened yogurt is rich in probiotics and can be a healthy add-in for dogs. It's particularly beneficial for dogs with digestive issues.

4. Grated Cheese: A sprinkle of grated cheese can make your dog's meal more enticing. Opt for low-fat varieties and use in moderation to avoid adding too many extra calories.

5. Fresh Herbs: Fresh herbs like parsley, basil, and oregano can add flavor and nutrients to your dog's meals. Parsley, in particular, is known for its breath-freshening properties.

6. Eggs: Cooked eggs (scrambled, boiled, or poached) are an excellent source of protein and can be mixed into your dog's meal for added nutrition. Be sure to cook eggs thoroughly to avoid the risk of salmonella.

7. Cooked Vegetables: Adding small amounts of cooked vegetables like peas, carrots, or green beans can provide extra vitamins and fiber. Make sure the vegetables are cooked until soft and cut into small pieces to avoid choking hazards.

8. Fruit: Small amounts of fresh fruit like blueberries, strawberries, or apples can add a touch of sweetness and antioxidants to your dog's meal. Always remove seeds and cores, and introduce new fruits gradually.

9. Coconut Oil: In addition to its health benefits, coconut oil can add a rich flavor to your dog's food. Mix a small amount into their meal for a taste that most dogs love.

10. Bone Broth Ice Cubes: Freeze bone broth in ice cube trays and add a cube or two to your dog's meal for a tasty, hydrating treat. This is especially refreshing in warm weather.

By incorporating these supplements and add-ins, you can enhance the nutritional value and appeal of your dog's meals. Whether you're addressing specific health concerns or simply want to give your dog a little something extra, these options allow you to tailor each meal to your dog's unique needs. Remember, always consult with your veterinarian before making significant changes to your dog's diet or introducing new supplements.

Feeding Tips and Storage

Proper feeding and storage practices are essential to ensure that your homemade dog food remains safe, fresh, and nutritious. This section will guide you through the best ways to store your dog's meals, portion their food, and transition them to homemade diets smoothly. By following these tips, you can ensure that your dog enjoys every meal while receiving the full benefits of the nutritious recipes you've prepared.

Proper Storage Techniques

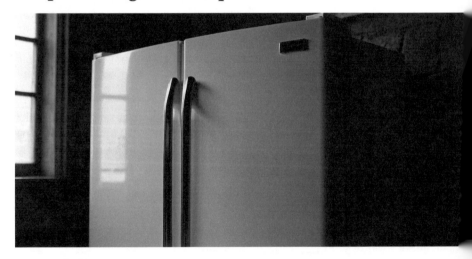

1. Refrigeration:

   - After cooking, allow the dog food to cool to room temperature befor transferring it to airtight containers. Properly sealed containers help pre vent contamination and maintain freshness.

   - Store the food in the refrigerator for up to 3-5 days. Make sure to label th containers with the date the food was prepared to keep track of freshnes

   - If you prepare large batches of food, consider dividing the meals int individual portions before refrigerating. This makes it easier to grab an serve at mealtime.

2. Freezing:

- For long-term storage, freezing is the best option. Divide the food into portion-sized containers or freezer-safe bags. Remove as much air as possible to prevent freezer burn.

- Store the food in the freezer for up to 2-3 months. Again, label each container with the preparation date to keep track of storage times.

- When you're ready to use frozen food, thaw it in the refrigerator overnight. Avoid thawing at room temperature, as this can lead to bacterial growth.

3. Portioning:

- Use portion-sized containers to store individual meals. This not only makes feeding more convenient but also helps in maintaining portion control.

- If you're unsure of the correct portion size for your dog, consult your veterinarian for guidance based on your dog's size, age, and activity level.

4. Reheating:

- When serving refrigerated or thawed food, you can lightly warm it to enhance its aroma and make it more appealing to your dog. However, avoid using a microwave, as it can create hot spots that might burn your dog's mouth.

- Instead, warm the food in a pan over low heat or place the container in warm water for a few minutes. Always check the temperature before serving to ensure it's not too hot.

Transitioning to Homemade Dog Food

Switching from commercial dog food to homemade meals can be a big change for your dog's digestive system. A gradual transition helps prevent digestive upset and allows your dog to adjust to the new diet smoothly.

1. Gradual Introduction:

- Start by mixing a small amount of homemade food into your dog's regular commercial food. A good ratio to begin with is 25% homemade food to 75% commercial food.

- Gradually increase the proportion of homemade food over 7-10 days. Move from 25% homemade to 50%, then to 75%, until you're feeding 100% homemade meals.

- Monitor your dog's response to the new food during this transition. Watch for any signs of digestive upset, such as vomiting, diarrhea, or changes in stool consistency. If your dog shows any signs of discomfort, slow down the transition process.

2. Consistency is Key:

- Dogs thrive on consistency, so try to keep the feeding schedule and portion sizes consistent once you've transitioned to homemade food.

- Feeding your dog at the same times each day helps regulate their digestive system and prevents overeating or begging between meals.

3. Monitoring Weight and Health:

- Regularly monitor your dog's weight, energy levels, and overall health after switching to homemade food. Significant weight loss, weight gain, or lethargy could indicate that the diet needs adjustment.

- Keep in touch with your veterinarian, especially during the initial months of feeding homemade food, to ensure that your dog is receiving the proper nutrition.

Portion Sizes and Feeding Schedules

Determining the right portion size and feeding schedule for your dog depends on several factors, including their age, size, activity level, and overall health. Below are some general guidelines, but it's always best to consult with your veterinarian for personalized advice.

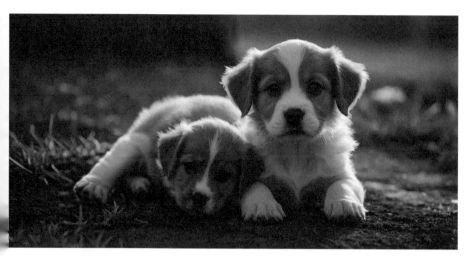

1. Puppies:

   ○ Portion Size: Puppies typically require more calories per pound of body weight than adult dogs because they are growing rapidly. Divide their daily food intake into 3-4 meals.

   ○ Feeding Schedule: Feed puppies 3-4 times per day at regular intervals. This helps maintain their energy levels and supports healthy growth.

2. Adult Dogs:

   ○ Portion Size: Adult dogs usually eat 2 meals per day. The portion size depends on their size, breed, and activity level. Active dogs may require more food, while less active dogs will need smaller portions.

   ○ Feeding Schedule: Most adult dogs do well with 2 meals per day, one in the morning and one in the evening. Try to stick to a consistent schedule to help with digestion and prevent overeating.

3. Senior Dogs:

   ○ Portion Size: Senior dogs may require fewer calories due to reduced activity levels. However, they still need nutrient-dense meals to maintain muscle mass and overall health.

- Feeding Schedule: Senior dogs may benefit from 2-3 smaller meals per day to help with digestion and prevent weight gain.

4. Special Cases:

- Overweight Dogs: If your dog needs to lose weight, reduce their portion sizes and focus on low-calorie, nutrient-rich foods. Consider dividing their daily food into smaller, more frequent meals to help them feel full.

- Underweight Dogs: If your dog needs to gain weight, increase their portion sizes slightly and include calorie-dense, but healthy, ingredients like lean meats, sweet potatoes, and healthy fats like coconut oil.

5. Using a Kitchen Scale:

- Weighing your dog's food with a kitchen scale can help ensure that you're feeding the correct portion size. This is especially important for weight management.

Monitoring Your Dog's Response

It's important to observe how your dog responds to their new homemade diet. Some key things to monitor include:

1. Energy Levels:

- Your dog's energy levels should remain stable or even improve on a homemade diet. If you notice a decrease in energy, it may indicate that your dog isn't getting enough calories or the right balance of nutrients.

2. Coat and Skin Health:

- A shiny coat and healthy skin are signs of good nutrition. If you notice any changes such as dry skin, dandruff, or a dull coat, it might be necessary to adjust the diet or add supplements like omega-3 fatty acids.

3. Stool Quality:

- Your dog's stool should be firm, well-formed, and consistent. Loose stools or diarrhea can indicate that the diet isn't agreeing with your dog, while hard, dry stools might suggest dehydration or too little fiber.

4. Weight:

- Regularly weigh your dog to ensure they are maintaining a healthy weight. Sudden weight loss or gain should be addressed by adjusting portion sizes or consulting with your veterinarian.

5. Appetite:

- A healthy dog should have a good appetite. If your dog becomes disinterested in their food, it may be due to a lack of flavor variety or an underlying health issue. Try adding some safe add-ins to boost flavor or consult your vet if the issue persists.

Handling Food Safety

Food safety is critical when preparing and storing homemade dog food. Here are some key tips to ensure your dog's food is safe to eat:

1. Hygiene:

   - Wash your hands thoroughly before and after handling dog food, especially raw meats. Use separate cutting boards and utensils for dog food preparation to prevent cross-contamination.

   - Clean all food preparation surfaces, utensils, and storage containers with hot, soapy water after use.

2. Cook Meat Thoroughly:

   - Ensure that all meat is cooked to a safe internal temperature to kill harmful bacteria. Use a meat thermometer to check the temperature if necessary.

   - Avoid feeding your dog raw or undercooked meat unless you are following a specific raw food diet plan recommended by your veterinarian.

3. Avoid Toxic Ingredients:

   - Some human foods are toxic to dogs, including onions, garlic, chocolate, grapes, raisins, and certain artificial sweeteners like xylitol. Ensure that these ingredients are never included in your dog's meals.

   - Be cautious with herbs and spices. While some, like parsley and turmeric, are beneficial, others can be harmful.

4. Storage Containers:

   - Use food-grade, airtight containers for storing homemade dog food. This helps keep the food fresh and prevents contamination.

   - Avoid using containers that have previously held human food with strong odors, as these can transfer to the dog food and affect its taste.

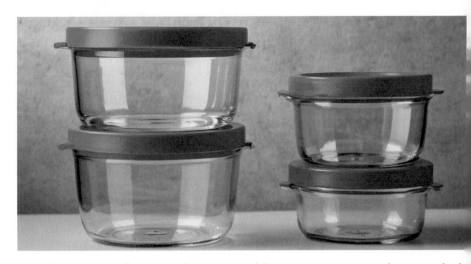

By following these feeding and storage guidelines, you can ensure that your dog's meals are safe, nutritious, and enjoyable. Proper storage extends the freshness of homemade food, while careful portioning and feeding schedules help maintain your dog's health and well-being. Regularly monitor your dog's response to their diet, and don't hesitate to make adjustments as needed to keep them happy and healthy.

Frequently Asked Questions

When it comes to homemade dog food, pet owners often have many questions about nutrition, safety, and the transition process. This section addresses some of the most common concerns and provides clear answers to help you feel confident in preparing and feeding your dog homemade meals.

1. Is homemade dog food better than commercial dog food?

Homemade dog food can offer several benefits over commercial dog food, including higher quality ingredients, no preservatives or fillers, and the ability to tailor meals to your dog's specific needs. However, homemade dog food requires careful planning to ensure it is nutritionally balanced. Commercial dog food is often formulated by experts to meet all nutritional requirements, which can be more convenient for some pet owners. Ultimately, the best choice depends on your dog's individual needs and your ability to provide a balanced homemade diet.

2. How do I know if my dog is getting all the nutrients they need?

Ensuring that your dog gets all the essential nutrients is critical when feeding homemade dog food. It's important to include a variety of ingredients to cover the full spectrum of nutrients, including proteins, fats, carbohydrates, vitamins, and minerals. Supplements can also be used to fill any gaps. Consulting with a veterinarian or a veterinary nutritionist is recommended, especially when first transitioning to homemade dog food. They can help you formulate balanced meals or recommend appropriate supplements.

3. How much homemade food should I feed my dog?

The amount of homemade food you should feed your dog depends on several factors, including their age, size, activity level, and overall health. A general guideline is to feed your dog about 2-3% of their ideal body weight in food per day. For example, a 50-pound dog might eat about 1-1.5 pounds of food daily. However, it's important to monitor your dog's weight and adjust portions as needed. Your veterinarian can provide specific recommendations based on your dog's individual needs.

4. Can I switch my dog to homemade food all at once?

It's generally recommended to transition your dog to homemade food gradually to avoid digestive upset. Start by mixing a small amount of homemade food with their current food and gradually increase the proportion of homemade food over 7-10 days.

This allows your dog's digestive system to adjust to the new diet. If your dog shows signs of digestive discomfort, such as vomiting or diarrhea, slow down the transition process.

5. What should I do if my dog doesn't like the homemade food?

If your dog is hesitant to eat homemade food, there are a few strategies you can try:

- Flavor Enhancers: Add low-sodium broth, a small amount of cheese, or some plain yogurt to make the food more appealing.

- Gradual Introduction: Mix the homemade food with their current food in small amounts until they get used to the new taste and texture.

- Texture Adjustments: Some dogs prefer different textures, so you can try pureeing the food or adding a bit of crunch with chopped vegetables or kibble.

If your dog still refuses the food, consult your veterinarian to rule out any underlying health issues or get further guidance.

6. Can I use the same recipes for puppies, adult dogs, and senior dogs?

While many ingredients can be used for dogs at all life stages, the proportions and nutritional needs vary depending on the dog's age. Puppies require more calories, protein, and certain nutrients to support growth, while senior dogs may need fewer calories but more joint-supporting nutrients like glucosamine. It's important to tailor the recipes to your dog's life stage or consult with a veterinarian to ensure that the meals meet your dog's specific nutritional requirements.

7. How often should I rotate the protein sources in my dog's diet?

Rotating protein sources can provide a wider range of nutrients and reduce the risk of developing food sensitivities. You can rotate proteins weekly, bi-weekly, or monthly depending on what works best for your dog. Common protein sources to rotate include chicken, turkey, beef, lamb, and fish. Make sure to introduce new protein gradually to avoid digestive issues.

8. Is it safe to add spices and herbs to my dog's food?

Some spices and herbs are safe and even beneficial for dogs, while others can be harmful. Safe herbs include parsley, basil, turmeric, and oregano, which can add flavor and provide health benefits like anti-inflammatory properties. However, avoid spices like garlic, onions, and large amounts of salt, as they can be toxic to dogs. Always research or consult with your veterinarian before adding new spices or herbs to your dog's food.

9. What if I need to travel? Can I still feed my dog homemade food?

Yes, you can still feed your dog homemade food while traveling. Here are some options:

- Freeze Ahead: Prepare and freeze individual portions of homemade food before your trip. You can thaw and serve as needed.

- Portable Containers: Store portions in airtight containers or resealable bags for easy transport. Keep them in a cooler if refrigeration isn't available.

- Combine with Commercial Food: If traveling long distances or for extended periods, you might combine homemade food with a high-quality commercial dog food to ensure your dog gets balanced meals.

10. What if I make a mistake in the recipe? Will it harm my dog?

Minor variations in recipes are usually not harmful as long as the main ingredients are safe for dogs and the meals remain nutritionally balanced. However, it's important to avoid toxic ingredients like onions, garlic, chocolate, and certain artificial sweeteners. If you're unsure about an ingredient or if your dog has eaten something potentially harmful, contact your veterinarian immediately. To minimize mistakes, follow recipes carefully and consult with a veterinarian if you have any concerns about ingredients or nutritional balance.

This FAQ section addresses common concerns and questions about feeding homemade dog food, providing you with the knowledge and confidence to make informed decisions about your dog's diet. If you have additional questions or specific concerns, don't hesitate to reach out to your veterinarian for personalized advice.

Heartfelt Dog Training – Preview

Chapter One - Navigating the Canine Mind - Understanding Your Dog's Behavior

1.1 Unraveling the Dog's Mind: Instincts, Emotions, and Cognition

Understanding the intricate workings of your dog's mind is the first step towards effective communication and training. A dog's mind is a fascinating blend of instincts, emotions, and cognitive abilities, each playing a unique role in shaping their behavior and interactions with the world around them.

Instincts: The Inborn Behaviors

Instincts are hardwired into your dog's DNA. They are the natural tendencies that guide behaviors like hunting, scavenging, mating, and even nurturing. For instance, you might notice your dog sniffing and tracking scents during a walk, or you may observe herding breeds trying to gather and move other animals or people - these are expressions of their instinctual behaviors.

Understanding these instincts is crucial because they can often explain certain behaviors that might otherwise be puzzling or frustrating. For example, a retriever might have an innate love for fetching objects, while a terrier could display a strong prey drive. Recognizing and respecting these instincts, and providing appropriate outlet for them, is key to a happy and mentally stimulated dog.

Emotions: The Feel of the Canine World

Dogs experience a range of emotions, much like humans do. They feel joy, fear, love, excitement, and even get stressed or anxious. These emotions can significantly impact their behavior. A dog wagging its tail exuberantly exhibits joy, while one with its tail tucked between its legs might be showing fear or anxiety.

Emotions in dogs are often more straightforward than in humans. They live in the moment and their emotions are usually a direct response to their immediate environment or experiences. This emotional transparency makes it easier for us to understand and respond to their needs. For example, recognizing signs of fear or stress in your dog is essential to avoid situations that make them uncomfortable and to provide reassurance and safety.

Cognition: The Thinking Dog

Cognition in dogs covers their learning abilities, memory, perception, problem-solving skills, and even their capacity for understanding human language and gestures. Dogs are intelligent creatures with a remarkable ability to learn from their environment and from their interactions with us.

A significant part of a dog's cognitive ability revolves around their social intelligence. Dogs are exceptionally skilled at reading human body language and can often understand our intentions and emotions better than we realize. This social cognition is what makes dogs such incredible companions. They can learn commands, follow instructions, and even anticipate our needs in some cases.

Training and mental stimulation play a vital role in keeping your dog's cognitive abilities sharp. Engaging them in activities that challenge their mind, like puzzle toys, obedience training, and new tricks, not only strengthens their mental faculties but also deepens the bond you share with them.

The Interplay of Instincts, Emotions, and Cognition

In training and everyday interactions, it's important to remember that a dog's behavior is often a complex mix of their instincts, emotions, and cognitive abilities. A dog might bark excessively (instinct) because it's anxious (emotion) or because it has learned that barking gets your attention (cognition).

Understanding this interplay helps us approach training and behavior modification in a holistic way. It allows us to provide outlets for instinctual behaviors, cater to their emotional needs, and engage their cognitive skills. This comprehensive understanding leads to a more empathetic and effective approach to training, ensuring a happier and well-adjusted dog.

The mind of a dog is a wondrous thing. By unraveling the complexities of their instincts, emotions, and cognition, we open the door to a deeper understanding and a stronger, more harmonious relationship. As we move forward in this book, we'll explore how these elements of the canine mind play out in different situations and how we can use this knowledge to enhance our training and our lives with our beloved canine companions.

Keep Reading and Get Your Copy Now!

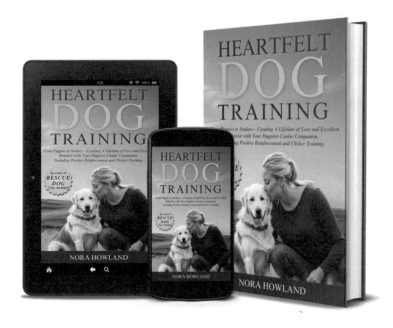

Made in the USA
Columbia, SC
07 December 2024

48698119R00048